Maxx Ketosis Guide

GLENIS GRAHAM

ISBN:9798541920758

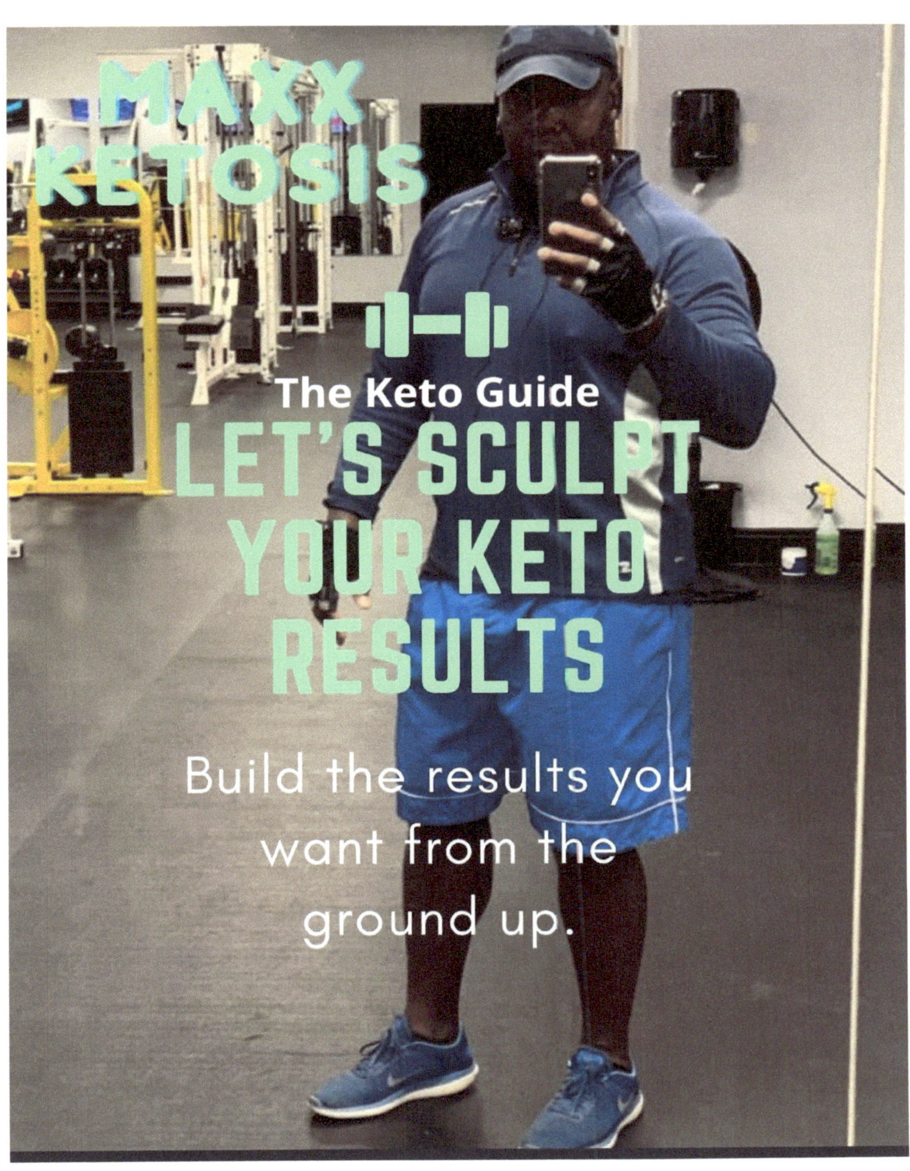
MAXX
KETOSIS
The Keto Guide
LET'S SCULPT
YOUR KETO
RESULTS
Build the results you
want from the
ground up.

Legal Disclaimer

The publisher and the author are providing this book and its contents on an "as is" basis and make no representations or warranties of any kind with respect to this book or its contents. The publisher and the author disclaim all such representations and warranties, including but not limited to warranties of healthcare for a particular purpose. In addition, the publisher and the author assume no responsibility for errors, inaccuracies, omissions, or any other inconsistencies herein.

The content of this book is for informational purposes only and is not intended to diagnose, treat, cure, or prevent any condition or disease. You understand that this book is not intended as a substitute for consultation with a licensed practitioner. Please consult with your own physician or healthcare specialist regarding the suggestions and recommendations made in this book. The use of this book implies your acceptance of this disclaimer.

The publisher and the author make no guarantees concerning the level of success you may experience by following the advice and strategies contained in this book, and you accept the risk that results will differ for each individual. The testimonials and examples provided in this book show exceptional results, which may not apply to the average reader, and are not intended to represent or guarantee that you will achieve the same or similar results.

Introduction

I'm can assume that if you're reading this Maxx Ketosis Guide you're very aware it's hard to stick to a diet. You have so much to deal with. Hunger and cravings, not to mention the expense, all come to mind when you think of the word diet. But the truth is, some that expensive diet food can be harming you. It's usually over-processed to the point that your body probably doesn't even recognize that it is food. Our bodies cannot digest it, and you have stomach issues, heartburn, and vacillate between constipation and diarrhea.

But, if you have a good plan, it's not hard to stick to at all. Let me say this, I really shouldn't refer to the ketosis process as a diet, if you do it correctly it's more of a lifestyle change. So let me explain to you what I mean by that. The goal is to get your body into ketosis which means that your burning fat and not carbs for fuel. This honestly is the way that our bodies are designed to function. It is only in the modern ages that we started processing our food and, in that process, we have eliminated fibers and the proteins as well as natural elements that are food requires for us to be truly satisfying and be nutritious. Many of the facts that I will cover in this guide is nothing new, these facts have been around since man needed food, so that's from the beginning of time.

My goal and hope are this guide will help you to accomplish your goals with the ketosis lifestyle.

Contents

What Is Ketosis and What Makes It Beneficial?

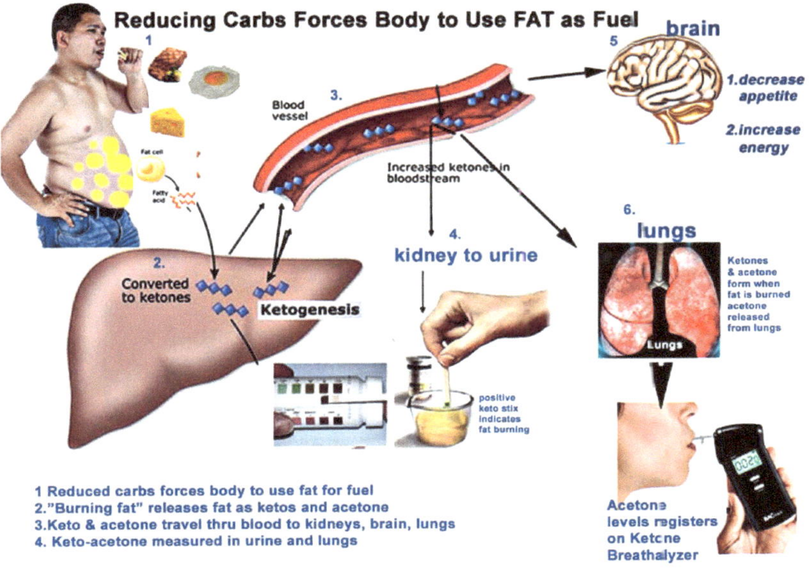

Maxx Ketosis is when you are in ketosis benefiting in a healthy life-changing way. Maxx Ketosis is a lifestyle change that consists of eating the ketogenic way: low carb, high healthy fat, and moderate protein 99 percent of the time - even if it's your birthday. What does it mean to eat ketogenic, though? Well, you eat in such a way that your body produces ketones. Don't worry, this is not scary; in fact, ketones can protect your brain from Alzheimer's and other problems, such as brain fog and memory.

What if you started eating the way your ancestors used to eat? What would that look like? When you consider what your ancestors did not have, namely processed food, you can see what that might look like. The food around was that which was easily available such as berries, wild animals, and vegetables that are easy to grow like spinach, cabbage, broccoli, and cauliflower.

Because it was hard to catch food, they also had to ensure everything they ate was as high in fat as possible so that they could keep on enough weight to be healthy. But not fake fat, of course - healthy fat from fruit like coconut oil and olive oil.

Some people also enjoy ghee, which is clarified butter, in this plan. That's the other thing that is awesome about the ketogenic lifestyle; you do have lots of leeway in what you eat if it follows the main goals, which are to eat low carb, high fat, and moderate protein most of the time.

Processed food is full of refined sugars, unhealthy fats, and chemicals that no one can pronounce and will leave you unsatisfied, always craving more. And guess what; it's not your fault if you're always craving more. They made the food that way.

The food you're eating is designed to cause cravings. Processed food is made to hook you on it, just like opiates. The food scientists know the exact combinations of fat, salt, and sugar to hook you. They've found the formula to make every meal into a drug. What's worse is that this drug will make you fat, unhealthy, prone to diabetes and you'll likely die earlier than you otherwise would. Even when you think you're eating small amounts of food called "diet" food, you can be fat and very unhealthy. Thin people who are eating a fully processed diet are also very unhealthy and prone to illness. The disease manifests differently in everyone.

Thankfully, the ketogenic diet has become more mainstream. People are taking to it and getting healthier. They're getting healthier because it's simple. They don't have to think too hard to know whether they can have that food or not. Due to this fact, it makes it easy for the ketogenic way of eating to become a full-on lifestyle.

That's good, because one thing that can ensure that people change for life, and make eating keto a habit, is to turn it into a lifestyle. When you know you're going to live this way forever, that you're not taking breaks, and that you're not doing it for just the next few weeks until the big party, then you tend to stick to a healthier way of eating because it's just normal and natural. Since ketogenetic eating is so natural, you'll agree that it can easily become a lifestyle.

Reasons the Ketogenic Lifestyle Is So Effective

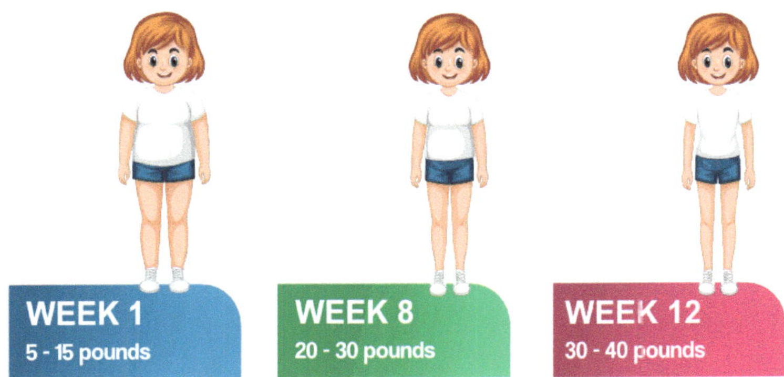

The main reason that the ketogenic lifestyle is so effective is simply that it works. When something you do gets results, it's easy to want to keep doing it. All you have to do is take the first steps, and after that, the proof is in the pudding.

It's Easy – Yes there are numerous products out today to make it easier still, but even if you never buy a single prepared item, it's still easy to eat this way. When you start doing it within a week, you'll realize that this is easier than what you did before.

You Don't Have to Spend Lots of Money – The keto lifestyle is simple and due to that it's not expensive, so you don't have to spend a lot of money. You can go out to almost any sit-down restaurant and find something to eat that will work, even if it's not perfect.

You Feel Satisfied – When you eat the right combination of food, you simply feel more satisfied. The food is higher in nutrition, so your body will eventually stop turning on the cravings because it's getting what it wants and needs. It doesn't hurt that the food is delicious.

You Feel More Energetic – Nothing is like the energy you get once your body has adjusted to the keto lifestyle, which will only take a few weeks of sticking to it. One day you'll wake up and feel so much more energetic, and because of that, you'll also be able to get more done in the 24 hours you're given.

Ends Brain Fog – You may not even know you have brain fog until it's cleared. When it clears, you'll wonder how you were surviving and getting things done before. You're going to feel so much clearer about everything.

Almost Everyone Can Do It – With few exceptions, almost anyone can eat this way. The main exception is someone with kidney disease. This is not because it's an unhealthy diet, but because someone with kidney disease must control their fluid intake and eat less protein.

You know it's true. When you do something that gives you pleasure, you keep doing it. We all make time for the things we really like doing, and once you get going on the ketogenic way of life, you'll want to keep going. You'll feel so much better fast that you'll be surprised. Don't test the waters and go back to your old ways, because you will find out that this lifestyle works.

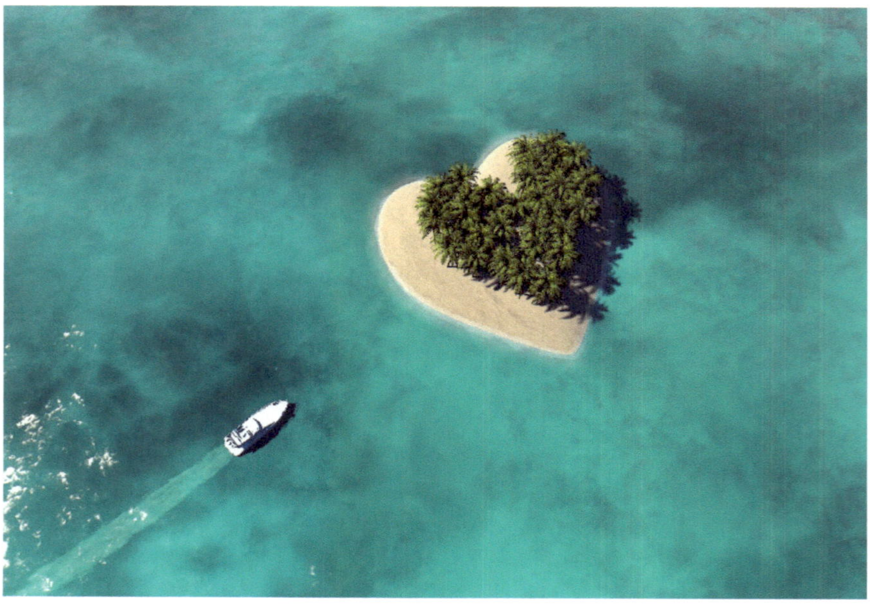

Other Benefits of the Ketogenic Lifestyle

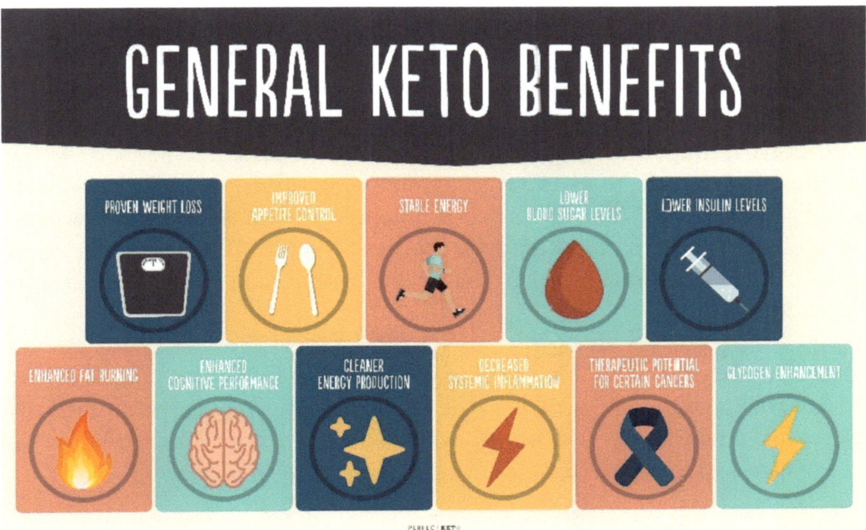

Besides being easy to stick to, there are enormous other benefits to the ketogenic lifestyle. It's amazing how well this way of eating works for improving and even reversing many diseases.

Fights Obesity – If you eat a ketogenic diet, eventually you will not be overweight. It's just a fact of life that eating keto properly will make you lose weight. At first, it'll happen fast and then it'll slow down, but if you're doing it, you'll be losing it.

Can Help Manage Diabetes – Keto lowers your blood sugar levels substantially since you will not be eating lots of high-starch veggies, lots of high-sugar fruit, or any processed food. In addition, you're going to be eating a variety of low-starch veggies, which is going to help you even further.

Can Improve Memory Issues – Because ketones are neuroprotective, some Alzheimer's patients have reported to show seen some improvements and slowing of the progression of the disease by maintaining a ketogenic lifestyle.

Potentially Can Helps Prevent / Slows Cancer – One of the most common types of brain cancer (gliomas) can shrink substantially in someone on a ketogenic diet. Going extra low carb and ensuring that you take out every single processed food will help with this.

Can Lowers High Blood Pressure – If you have high blood pressure, you may end up going off your meds after a few weeks of the keto way of life. Because the diet is anti-inflammatory, it helps to lower blood pressure.

Fights Chronic Inflammation – This way of life, drinking plenty of water, avoiding processed food, and eating enough nutrition, will keep your inflammation at bay. This is one reason people with autoimmune illness do so well on a keto way of life. Because you're not triggering your inflammatory response by what you're eating now, you won't get inflamed as much.

Can Be Helpful with Other Brain Disorders – Because ketones are neuroprotective, people with any type of brain issue - ranging from memory issues and brain fog to serious issues like stroke - will find that this way of eating can help improve their condition.

Improves Epilepsy – This has been a way of life for many people with intractable epilepsy, providing relief to many parents of children with epilepsy. Ketogenesis is featured in the movie about a child with epilepsy called Lorenzo's Oil, which is still very interesting to watch.

Can Help Reverse Polycystic Ovary Syndrome – A major cause of infertility today, the main reason people have PCOS is that they have elevated insulin levels. The high insulin environment will cause the ovaries to produce more male hormones called androgens, which can affect everything about this system. The keto way of eating can reverse this condition and if done soon enough will help restore fertility.

Can Reduce Migraines – Many people who live the ketogenic lifestyle report that they get many fewer migraines than they did before. It is thought that it works because the ketones are neuroprotective but also because of the reduction in inflammation.

The health benefits are so numerous that you can probably add to this list yourself once you get started. Many people report life-changing results from following the ketogenic lifestyle.

Eating Do's and Don'ts

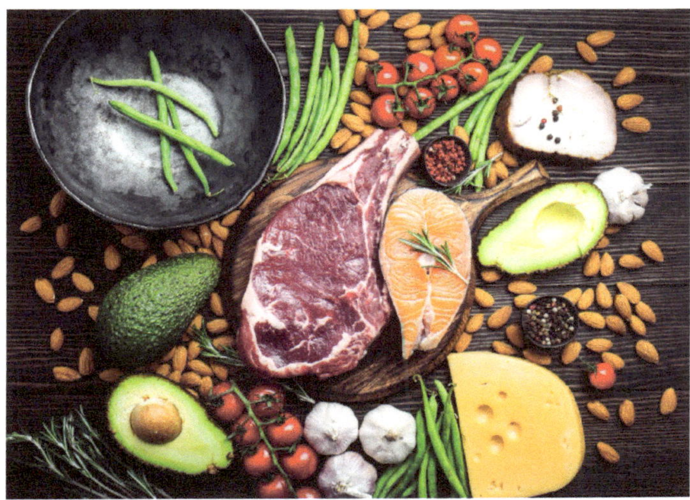

One thing that can help you find out more about this lifestyle is learning some eating dos and don'ts. This will make all the difference in your ability to turn this into your lifestyle. Because here's the thing; if you're following a lifestyle, you cannot put your toe in another lifestyle every day and expect to see results. Therefore, if you want to follow this way of life, study this list.

Don't Eat High Protein – The ketogenic way of eating is not meant to be high protein. It's a high-fat diet but low in carbs and moderate in protein. You want to eat at least 60 percent of your calories in fat (can go up to 75 percent), only 15 to 30% from protein, and the rest up to 10 percent as carbs.

Do Choose the Right Type of Meat – The meat you choose should be as natural as possible. Don't buy meat that has been doctored with sugar and additives to make it taste better. You want to find organic, grass-fed, free-range, and so forth. However, just do the best you can and don't stress too much.

Do Eat Fruit Fats – The main fats that you want to eat should be natural. They should mostly come from fruit like olive oil and coconut oil. You can also use animal fats and ghee, but most of your fat should come from fruit.

Do Eat When Hungry – You don't need to restrict your food intake when you're eating keto. You can eat when you're hungry if it meets the rules of the ratio you're trying to stick to.

Don't Drink Milk – While you can have some dairy, living the ketogenic way you want to avoid drinking milk as a beverage. If you use any, a splash in your coffee is all you should use. One glass of milk can have quite a lot of carbs. Read your labels.

Don't Eat Sugar – This is the hardest part to get used to, but you will, and you'll be glad you did. But you cannot eat sugar, and you should try to avoid adding any type of sweetener to any of your food for a few weeks. Later you can use some sweeteners if you must, such as stevia.

Do Drink Your Bone Broth – One thing that some people overlook is the bone broth. Drinking it is your key to sticking to this long enough that it becomes second nature and finally a true lifestyle for you.

Do Enjoy Something Special – On special occasions, you won't ruin everything if you enjoy a glass of dry wine, whiskey, brandy, vodka or any low-sugar drink of your choice and a serving of at least 70% dark chocolate. Count your carbs, and you can do it at least weekly.

Eating right on the ketogenic way of life is not hard to do. If you can visually divide your plate to fit the food on it in the right quantities, that will help. They even sell some keto plates online; just do a Google search to find out more. here.

Common Side Effects and How to Combat Them

Many people call the combination of symptoms they have when first embarking on the keto way as the "keto flu." If you do feel any of these symptoms and side effects, realize that they are just a sign that you're pushing your body into ketosis. Once the change fully occurs, you'll start feeling better.

These unpleasant side effects may include:

- Headache
- Fatigue
- Moodiness
- Brain fog
- Unmotivated
- Vertigo
- Cravings
- Nausea
- Muscle cramps
- Constipation
- Keto breath
- Heart palpitations

How to Combat Side Effects

Drink More Water - Pretty much every single symptom you get can be combated by ensuring that you are properly hydrated. Try drinking more of your bone broth during the day and drinking 32 ounces of water with citrus every morning. It may also help you to measure out your water, so you know you're drinking enough.

Check Your Ratios – Are you keeping your fat ratio high and your carbs low? If you tend to fall off the wagon every weekend or monthly, you're going to cause your body to struggle harder. If you feel like you're sticking to everything, go back to checking ratios to be sure.

Boost Your Carb Intake – If you have suffered more than a couple of weeks without getting relief, you may want to add more carbs. But let's be clear, by carbs we mean that you should eat more veggies. Try upping your veggies for a couple of weeks to see if that helps.

Work Out Carefully – When you're in transition, it's okay to baby yourself and do slower and more gentle forms of exercise like walking, stretching, and swimming. Avoid strenuous exercise for at least the first month; after that, you'll likely be able to outperform your previous efforts.

Avoid Restricting Food Intake – If you get hungry, try to judge realistically whether you should eat something or not. If it's an hour before dinner, you're supposed to be hungry, so wait. But if it's more than that, it's okay to eat something small to take away the hunger. Don't focus on calories; only pay attention to your hunger.

Check Your Meds – Often people get to stop taking their meds when on the keto way of eating. If you notice anything that concerns you about your meds, talk to your doctor right away so they can advise you.

You can use breath spray in the meantime, but if you add more water, that will help too. Also, ensure that you're getting enough bone broth and eating in the right ratios without shocking your body. Don't allow cheat days every other day or week or month either. If you follow these guidelines, you'll find that these side effects go away on their own not to return - unless you kick your body out of ketosis and then back in by not minding your ratios.

Note: If you get heart palpitations, please do talk to your doctor about it - especially if you have diabetes.

Reasons to Stop or Modify Your Ketogenic Lifestyle

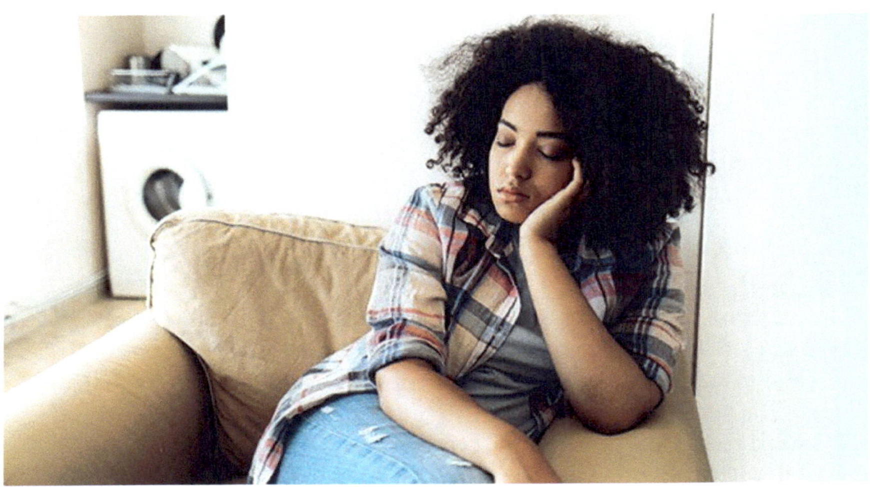

The strange fact about being a human is that as much as we're the same, we're all different. Everyone does not respond the same. Two different people can respond differently to a medication, a diet, or really anything. You're unique. Therefore, there are sometimes reasons to modify the keto lifestyle to fit your needs better.

Seizures – The keto diet that treats seizures is high fat, but low in carbs and low in protein. If you want to use the ketogenic lifestyle to treat something like that you should also speak to a physician who is trained in planning this type of diet.

Ketoacidosis – **Diabetic ketoacidosis** is a serious complication of diabetes that occurs when your body produces high levels of blood acids called ketones.

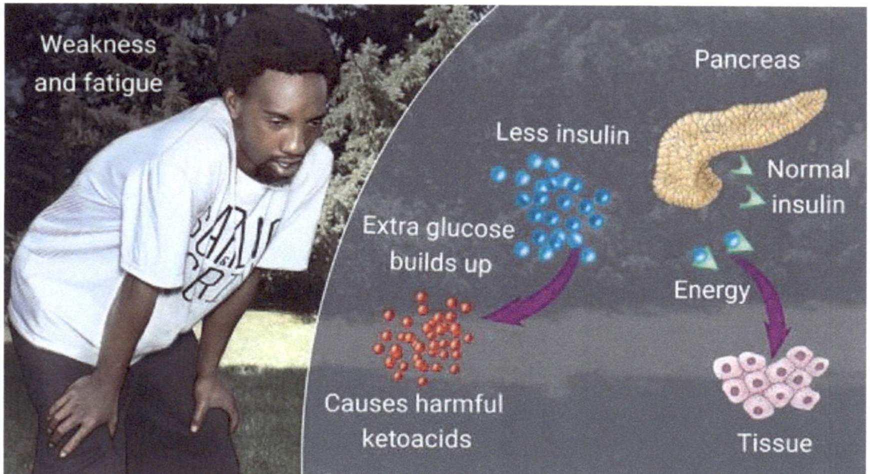

This is a serious diabetes complication where the body produces excess blood acids (ketones). This type of condition occurs when there is not sufficient insulin in the body. It can be triggered by infection or other illness. The **symptoms** will include thirst, frequent urination, some nausea, abdominal pain, weakness, fruity-scented breath, and confusion. The recovery will require hospital treatment to replace fluids and electrolytes and provide insulin therapy may also be needed.

Pregnancy – If you are pregnant, you can still enjoy the ketogenic lifestyle if you're ensuring you are getting enough nutrients. You don't want to lose weight, so boost your caloric intake by adding more fruit and more vegetables to your day and go ahead and add some nuts, seeds, legumes, and even some dairy.

Losing Too Much Weight – Once you get to your normal weight, it can be a challenge to figure out how much food to add. Always add in more veggies and fruit and see if you can add more varieties of food in small amounts from the nuts, seed, and legume category too.

You Work Out a Lot – If you work out a lot and are losing weight using keto, you may experience muscle cramps after or during your workouts. Consider adding some fast-digesting carbs before your workout to help.

You Simply Feel Bad – If you've given it a go for at least a month and you still do not feel good about this lifestyle, you should stop. But you should also go to the doctor to get a full check-up in case there is an underlying illness you're missing.

You're a Body Builder – If you're a bodybuilder, you may need to eat a lot more carbs. You may even be able to do this without affecting whether you're in ketosis or not.

You Are Diagnosed with Kidney Disease – You may need to lower your protein further if you are diagnosed with kidney disease. However, that doesn't mean you have to quit; just modify.

You Take Medication – You may need to slow your transition to ketosis if you're using certain meds, especially insulin and blood pressure medication. If you're having issues, just go more slowly with moving down your carbs and upping your fat.

Having Trouble Getting into Ketosis – Some people are resistant, and it will take more work to get into ketosis. You may have to lower your carbs even more than normal at first. Check ingredients on everything to ensure you're not getting added sugars you didn't know about; this is often the case as sugar is used in a lot of meat preparations.

Bonus Note Tip: If you are having trouble getting into ketosis there is one drink that I know can assist you with the whole ketosis process and works with any type of diet or lifestyle you follow. More importantly this drink can get ketones in your system fast. Get the all the details:
http://gmaxx.DrinkYourSample.com

There is never a real reason to quit the ketogenic lifestyle. You can change your ratios of fat, carbs, and protein around if you keep it within the ranges discussed before. When you do adjust your levels, don't reach for the processed food that you're not supposed to have. Instead, reach for healthy additions to your plate.

Common Questions about the Ketogenic Lifestyle

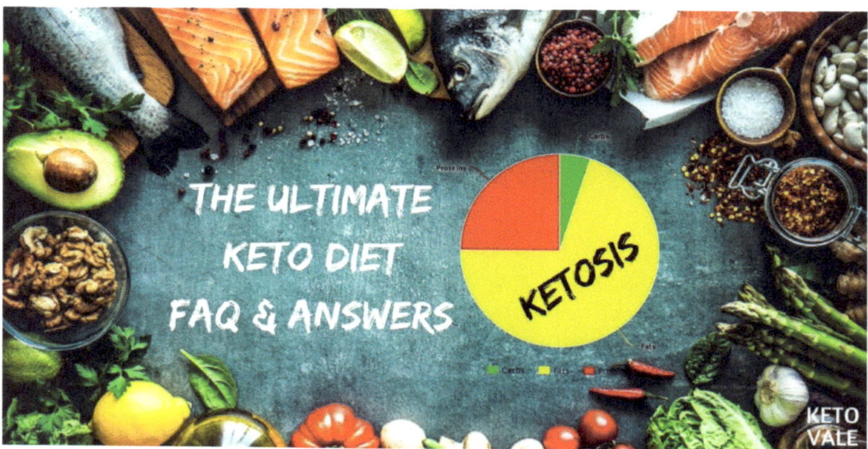

The ketogenic way of life is very safe if you're doing it correctly, putting nutrition above everything else. But like most situations, everyone wants something for nothing. The ketogenic lifestyle is not about eating a pound of bacon every day; in fact, that would not be good for anyone to do at all.

Here are answers to some common questions about the keto lifestyle.

Should I Talk to My Doctor?

Most people can do it easily and successfully with only good things to report. However, almost everyone can benefit from seeing their doctor before starting a diet. This is especially true for anyone who is taking medication for diseases like diabetes and high blood pressure. This is because this diet is very powerful, and you will lower your blood pressure and blood sugar levels. How much depends on the person.

Some doctors don't like any type of "diet" and others are partial to other types of "diets." There is a lot of opinions that go into doctoring, so don't take it personally. The first question you want to ask your doctor is how they feel about the keto lifestyle or a low-carb diet in general. Then you may want to ask follow-up questions based on their answer.

If they do know about the real keto lifestyle, you can then ask any other questions you may have. Write them down before you go so that you don't forget. It's easy to feel rushed in the doctor's office. A good thing to ask for is "before" tests to find out where you stand health-wise; you can then get a check-up in a couple of months to see how well you're doing.

What Food Can I Eat on the Keto Lifestyle?

In general, you want to ensure you eat the right ratio of fat, carbohydrates, and protein. Most people will be in the following ranges: 60 to 75% calories from fat, 15 to 30% calories from protein and 5 to 10% from carbohydrates.

To fill those macronutrient ratios, you'll need to eat only whole healthy food that is produced in the most natural way possible, without the use of hormones and chemicals. Plus, you should not eat any processed food.

This is a healthy lifestyle. Just because something is "low carb" or says "keto" on it, doesn't mean it's good for you. What you will eat are healthy sources of protein in moderate amounts, fresh veggies of all sorts, some fruit, and healthy fat. Most of your calories are supposed to come from healthy fats from sources like coconut, olive, nuts, and seeds. When you have a choice, always eat the whole thing over going for the processed version. For example, eating olives gives you healthy olive fat plus veggie nutrients.

What Should I Not Eat on the Keto Lifestyle?

This is a short and easy answer because there isn't much you cannot eat when you think about it. Compare it to other lifestyles, and you quickly realize that every single healthy way of eating includes avoiding processed food, sugar, salt, and unhealthy fats - especially in combination. When you live the ketogenic lifestyle, it's easy to say no because you realize those things aren't food. There is no world where eating pop tarts for breakfast, for instance, is going to be healthy.

The foods you should not eat on keto are:

- Flour
- Grains
- Most fruit
- Refined Sugars
- Soft Drinks/Fruit Juices
- Starchy Vegetables

You can literally eat everything else. Name one diet where you can eat the things on this list in a way that you want to eat them. No one wants to eat whole grains without fat on them, but that's the only way you can eat them on that lifestyle and be healthy.

There are versions of some of these that you can make but remember that when you try to make something to take the place of something else, it never tastes as good. Instead, consider cooking new things that have their own special flavors that you enjoy. When you start reading labels, understand that if the ingredients include any of the above you should not eat it.

FOODS TO AVOID

GRAINS

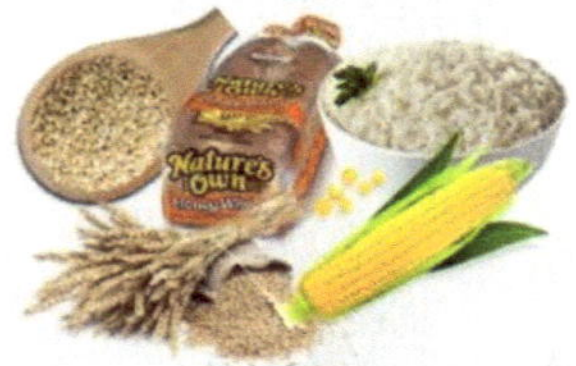

SUGARS

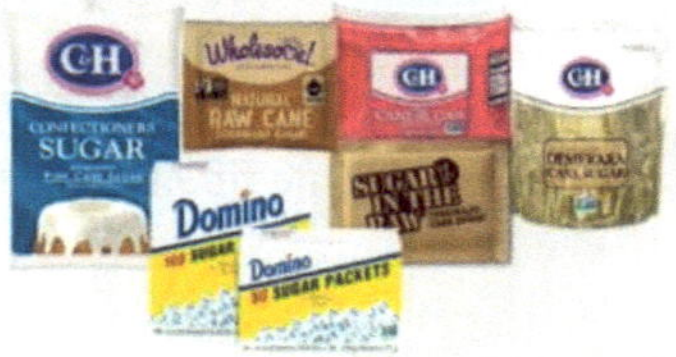

CALORIC BEVERAGES

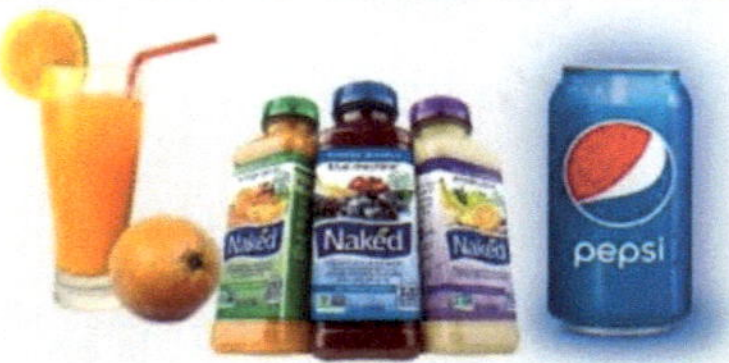

PROCESSED FOODS

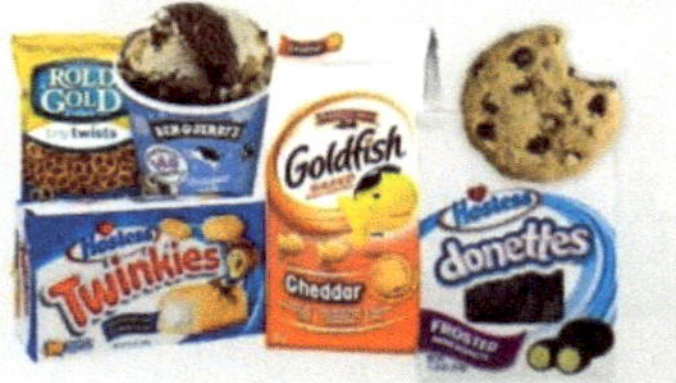

Do I Have to Count Calories?

Even though there are guidelines in terms of the ratios of the macronutrients that you eat, you don't have to count. You can just eyeball your meals on your plate. In general, a serving size of a piece of protein is the same size as the palm of your hand.

Fill your plate halfway with veggies, about a fourth of the plate should have the protein, and the rest of the plate includes all the fat you're supposed to eat - which of course is likely used to flavor the veggies and protein. Eat when you're hungry and stop when you're full. It is that easy. That is why it's such a good lifestyle.

However, if you want to, you can count calories when you first start. Start by eating at the top of the calorie requirements for your desired weight range and stay there if you're happy with the results. If you need to cut back more, you're at the top so you can still cut back.

You can also choose to figure out how many grams of carbohydrates would be in your ideal day and just count that, as this can often be simpler to keep track. As you grow into the lifestyle, you'll end up not needing to this, but in the beginning, it does help to know what you should be eating so you have an idea and guideline to go by.

Do I Need to Take Supplements?

Because of the state of our food sources, most people do need to take some supplements, but not as many as you might think. Remember, each person is very different, so the best thing to do is to look at your situation and find the right supplements for you.

So, in most cases, most of us can benefit from supplementing with MCT oil, BHB salts, vitamin B12, and vitamin D3. It's a great idea to ask your doctor for a blood test to determine your levels. The main problem with B12 and D3 is environmental. One of the inserting facts is we wash our food far too much to get enough B12, and some people just don't produce it, so almost everyone can benefit from taking a supplement for B12.

Apparently, the challenge with B12 is that a deficiency may not show up until it's way too late and it's irreversible and can cause serious neurological problems and major fatigue. The issue with vitamin D is that most people tend to wear sunscreen for good reason (and we should) and wash too (you should not wash for 24 to 48 hours after sun exposure to get enough D, but we feel icky and want to get the crud off). Having a vitamin D deficiency can result in body pain, lower back pain, and again cause fatigue.

Am I Going to Get High Cholesterol?

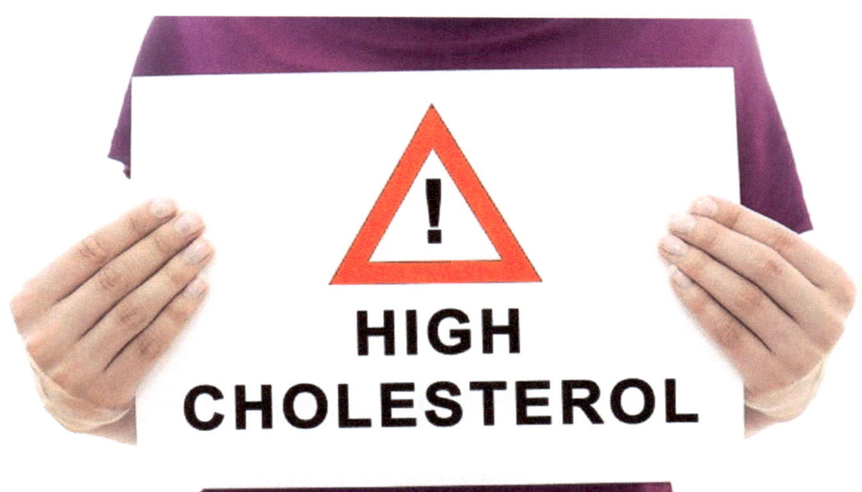

While no one can speak to how any lifestyle will affect another, research shows that the opposite happens to most people. Many people end up with higher-good cholesterol and lower bad cholesterol. The truth is, many people have high cholesterol due to genetics. The best thing to do is to get tested before, during, and after about 90 days of sticking to the ketogenic lifestyle. You may be surprised by the results, and so will your doctor.

Complete Keto Diet Food List

Complete Keto Diet Food List:
What You Can and Cannot Eat If You're on a Ketogenic Diet
Make eating keto a lot easier with this comprehensive keto diet food list—plus learn if it's the right diet for you.

The ketogenic diet is a high-fat, moderate-protein and very low-carbohydrate diet. Carbohydrates are the body's preferred source of energy, but on a strict ketogenic diet, less than 5 percent of energy intake is from carbohydrates. The reduction of carbohydrates puts the body into a metabolic state called ketosis. Ketosis is when the body starts breaking down stored fat into molecules called ketone bodies to use for energy, in the absence of circulating blood sugar from food. Once the body reaches ketosis, most cells will use ketone bodies to generate energy until you start eating carbohydrates again.

Traditionally, the ketogenic diet was only used in clinical settings to reduce seizures in children with epilepsy. "Now there is a lot of interest in the diet's effectiveness in helping with other neurological conditions, cancer, diabetes, PCOS [polycystic ovary syndrome], obesity, high cholesterol and cardiovascular disease," says Emily Stone, M.S., R.D. People also eat keto to lose weight.

Even if you know that you need to eat a very low-carb, high-fat, moderate protein diet—it can be confusing to know which foods to eat. This Maxx Ketosis Guide is very specific to foods you can eat, foods you should avoid and foods you can sometimes have when you're following a ketogenic diet.

Foods You Can Eat on the Ketogenic Diet

Here is a list of all the low-carb, keto-friendly foods that are appropriate to eat when you're following keto.

- Fish and seafood
- Low-carb veggies
- Cheese
- Avocados
- poultry
- Eggs
- Nuts, seeds and healthful oils
- Plain Greek yogurt and cottage cheese
- Berries
- Unsweetened coffee and tea
- Dark chocolate and cocoa powder

Fish and Seafood

Fish is rich in B vitamins, potassium, and selenium; it's also protein-rich and carb-free. Salmon, sardines, mackerel, albacore tuna and other fatty fish boast high levels of omega-3 fats, which have been found to lower blood sugar levels and increase insulin sensitivity. Frequent fish intake has been linked to a decreased risk of chronic disease as well as improved mental health. Aim to consume at least two 3-ounce servings of fatty fish weekly.

Low-Carb Veggies

Non-starchy vegetables are low in calories and carbs, but high in many nutrients, including vitamin C and several minerals. They also contain antioxidants that help protect against cell-damaging free radicals. Aim for non-starchy vegetables with less than 8 g of net carbs per cup. Net carbs are total carbohydrates minus fiber. Broccoli, cauliflower, green beans, bell peppers, zucchini and spinach fit the bill.

Cheese

Cheese has zero carbohydrates and is high in fat, making it a great fit for the ketogenic diet. It's also rich in protein and calcium. But, a 1-ounce slice of cheese delivers about 30 percent of the daily value for saturated fat, so if you're worried about heart disease consider portions when noshing on cheese.

Plain Greek Yogurt and Cottage Cheese

Yogurt and cottage cheese are high in protein and calcium-rich. Five ounces of plain Greek yogurt provides just 5 g of carbohydrates and 12 grams of protein. The same amount of cottage cheese also has 5 grams of carbohydrates with 18 grams of protein. Studies have shown that both calcium and protein can reduce appetite and promote fullness. Higher-fat yogurts and cottage cheese help keep you full for longer, and full-fat products would be part of the ketogenic diet.

Avocados

Choose heart-healthy fats like avocados, which are high in monounsaturated fat and potassium, a mineral many Americans are lacking. Half of a medium avocado contains 9 grams of total carbohydrates, 7 grams of which are fiber. Swapping animal fats for plant fats like avocados can help improve cholesterol and triglyceride levels.

Meat and Poultry

Meat is a source of lean protein and is considered a staple on the ketogenic diet. Fresh meat and poultry contain no carbohydrates and are rich in B vitamins and several minerals, including potassium, selenium and zinc. While processed meats, like bacon and sausage, are allowed on keto, they aren't the best for your heart and may raise your risk of certain types of cancer if you eat too much. Choose chicken, fish and beef more often and limit processed meats.

Eggs

Eggs are high in protein, B vitamins, minerals and antioxidants. Two eggs contain zero carbohydrates and 12 grams of protein. Eggs have been shown to trigger hormones that increase feelings of fullness and keep blood sugar levels stable, and they also contain antioxidants such as lutein and zeaxanthin, which help protect eye health.

Nuts, Seeds and Healthy Oils

Nuts and seeds are full of healthy polyunsaturated and monounsaturated fats, fiber and protein. They also are very low in net carbs. Olive oil and coconut oil are the two oils recommended on the keto diet. Olive oil is high in oleic acid and is associated with a lower risk of heart disease. Coconut oil is high in saturated fat but contains medium-chain triglycerides (MCTs), which can increase ketone production. MCTs may increase metabolic rate and promote the loss of weight and belly fat too. Measure portion sizes when consuming any type of healthy fat.

Carb counts for 1 oz. (28 g) of nuts and seeds (net carbohydrate equals total carbs minus fiber):

Almonds:	3 g net carbs (6 g total carbs)
Brazil nuts:	1 g net carbs (3 g total carbs)
Cashews:	8 g net carbs (9 g total carbs)
Macadamia nuts:	2 g net carbs (4 g total carbs)

Pecans:	1 g net carbs (4 g total carbs)
Pistachios:	5 g net carbs (8 g total carbs)
Walnuts:	2 g net carbs (4 g total carbs)
Chia seeds:	2 g net carbs (12 g total carbs)
Flaxseeds:	0 g net carbs (8 g total carbs)
Pumpkin seeds:	2 g net carbs (4 g total carbs)
Sesame seeds:	4 g net carbs (7 g total carbs)

Berries

Berries are rich in antioxidants that reduce inflammation and protect against disease. They are low in carbs and high in fiber.

Carb counts for 1/2 cup of some berries:

Blackberries:	3 g net carbs (7 g total carbs)
Blueberries:	9 g net carbs (11 g total carbs)
Raspberries:	3 g net carbs (7 g total carbs)
Strawberries:	3 g net carbs (6 g total carbs)

Unsweetened Coffee and Tea

Plain coffee and tea contain zero grams of carbohydrates, fat or protein, so they are A-OK on the keto diet. Studies show coffee lowers the risk of cardiovascular disease and type 2 diabetes. Tea is rich in antioxidants and has less caffeine than coffee; drinking tea may reduce the risk of heart attack and stroke, help with weight loss and boost your immune system.

Dark Chocolate and Cocoa Powder

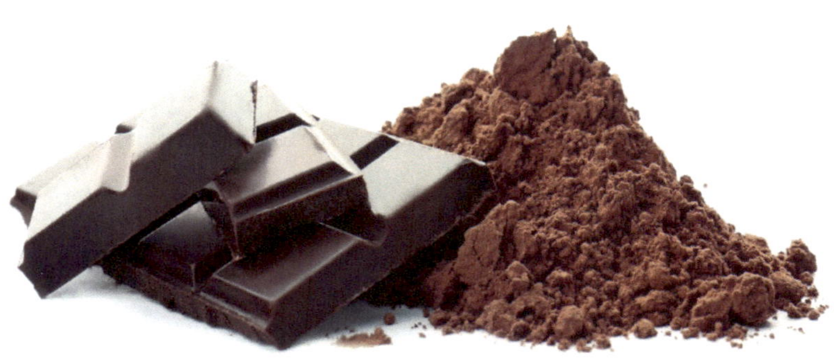

Check the label on these, as the amount of carbs depends on the type and how much you consume. Cocoa has been called a "superfruit" because it is rich in antioxidants, and dark chocolate contains flavanols, which may reduce the risk of heart disease by lowering blood pressure and keeping arteries healthy.

HEALTH BENEFITS OF
DARK CHOCOLATE

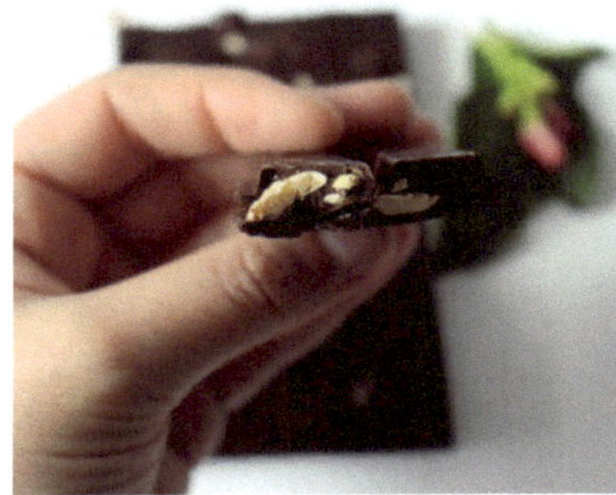

- High in: Potassium, Copper, Magnesium and Iron
- Increases blood flow in the brain
- May lower blood pressure
- May reduce risk for stroke
- High in Antioxidants
- Helps control blood sugar
- Improved mood

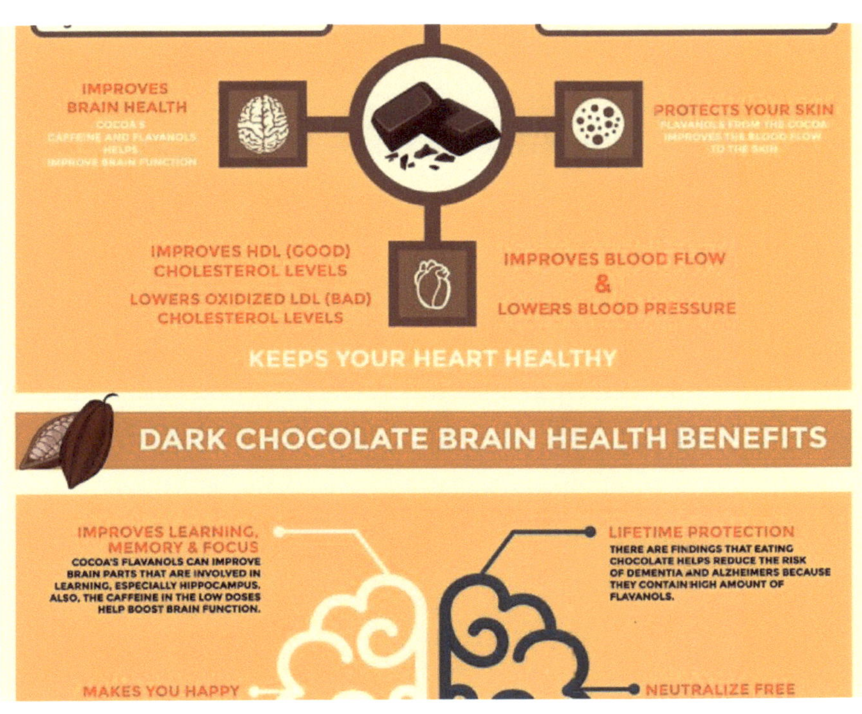

Can't Eat on the Keto Diet

List of Foods You Can't Eat on the Keto Diet:
- Grains
- Starchy vegetables and high-sugar fruits
- Sweetened yogurt
- Juices
- Honey, syrup or sugar in any form
- Chips and crackers
- Baked goods including gluten-free baked goods

Don't get too discouraged. Dietitians Stone and Laura Dority, M.S., R.D., L.D., with Keto Knowledge LLC, say that no foods are really off-limits on the keto diet. It's about total carbohydrate intake and how you choose to "spend" your carbs. Generally, you should stay under 20-40 grams of carbohydrates per day. "The exact amount needed to achieve ketosis can vary on the individual, though, with carb prescriptions ranging from 10 to 60 grams per day. This total is for net carbohydrates (total carbs minus fiber)," says Stone.

Dority adds, "Individuals who are really active can eat more carbs (maybe more at the 40-gram level) than someone who is sedentary."

High-Carb Foods That Most People Avoid on the Keto Diet

Grains

Cereal, crackers, rice, pasta, bread and beer are high in carbohydrates. Even whole-wheat pasta and the new bean-based pastas are high in carbs. Consider alternatives like spiralized vegetables or shirataki noodles, which are healthier low-carb options. Sugary breakfast cereals and healthy whole-grain cereals are high in carbohydrates too and should be avoided or minimized. "A slice of bread is 11 grams of carbs on average so technically you could have one slice a day maybe but that's spending all your carbs on pretty poor nutrition so I wouldn't recommend it when for the same carbs you could have A LOT of veggies," says Dority.

Alcohol Beer, and Wine

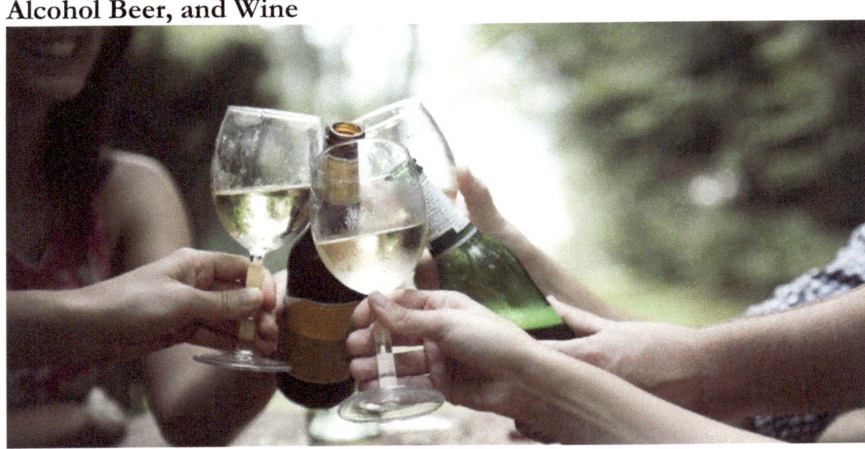

Beer can be enjoyed in moderation on a low-carb diet. Dry wine and spirits are better options, but all alcohol should be very limited.

Starchy vegetables and high-sugar fruits

Starchy vegetables contain more digestible carbohydrates than fiber and should be limited on the ketogenic diet. These include corn, potatoes, sweet potatoes and beets. Limit high-sugar fruits too, which spike your blood sugar more quickly than berries and have more.

Carb counts for high-sugar fruits:
Banana (1 medium):	24 g net carbs (27 g total carbs)
Raisins (1 oz. / 28 g):	21 g net carbs (22 g total carbs)
Dates (2 large):	32 g net carbs (36 g total carbs)
Mango (1 cup, sliced):	22 g net carbs (25 g total carbs)
Pear (1 medium):	21 g net carbs (27 g total carbs)

Carb counts for starchy vegetables:
Corn (1 cup):	32 g net carbs (36 g total carbs)
Potato (1 medium):	33 g net carbs (37 g total carbs)
Sweet potato (1 medium):	20 g net carbs (24 g total carbs)
Beets (1 cup, cooked):	14 g net carbs (17 g total carbs)

Sweetened yogurts

Stick to plain yogurt to limit added sugars (aka carbohydrates). Greek yogurt is higher in protein and lower in carbohydrates compared to regular yogurt.

Juices

Fruit juice-natural or not-is high in fast-digesting carbs that spike your blood sugar. Stick to water.

Honey, syrup and sugar in any form

Avoid sugar, honey, maple syrup and other forms of sugar, which are high in carbohydrates and low in nutrients.

Chips and crackers

Avoid chips, crackers and other processed, grain-based snack foods, which are high in carbohydrates and low in fiber.

Gluten-free baked goods

Gluten-free does not equal carb-free. In fact, many gluten-free breads and muffins are as high in carbohydrates as traditional baked goods. They usually lack fiber too.

Foods and Drinks You Can Sometimes Have on the Keto Diet

You can technically have any food on the keto diet if it falls within your daily carbohydrate goal, but these foods fall in the middle between high-carb and low-carb.

Milk

Milk is an excellent source of calcium, potassium and several B vitamins. But, 1 cup has 12 grams of sugar (lactose). Choose almond, coconut or another low-carb milk instead.

Beans and Legumes

Beans and legumes are high in fiber and protein and are part of a heart-healthy diet but are also high in carbohydrates. They may be included in small amounts on a ketogenic diet. However, it's often recommended to avoid them altogether.

BEANS AND LEGUMES

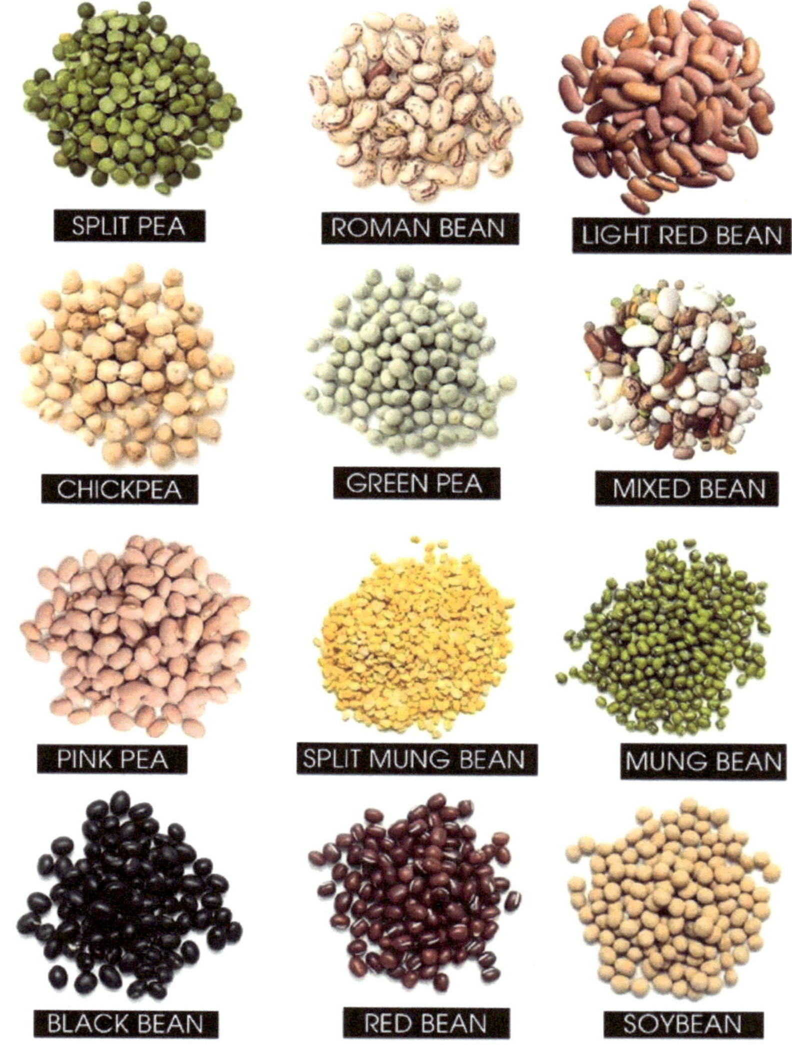

Pros of the Ketogenic Diet

"There is solid evidence to support use of the ketogenic diet in individuals with epilepsy who have seizures that are drug resistant," says Dority. In the short term, people who follow the diet report weight loss. Dority says, "There is certainly some good recent research showing promise in disorders such as autism, traumatic brain injury, brain tumors, migraines and Alzheimer's (to name a few but the list could go on), as well as some great research on ketogenic diets and type 2 diabetes reversal including dramatically reducing insulin needs, fasting blood sugar levels, lowering A1C and obtaining significant weight loss."

Cons of the Ketogenic Diet

"Like most highly restrictive diets, it is difficult to meet nutritional needs while doing keto," says Stone. "It often comes with uncomfortable side effects like constipation and the 'keto flu.' Also, the long-term health consequences are not well understood.

Take Away

We've discussed what makes the ketogenic way of eating so effective, the health benefits, and why it's a great lifestyle to be part of. We've also covered what to eat and what not to eat, the side effects of eating this way, and how to make it your lifestyle easily. Finally, we've given some common questions and answers about the ketogenic lifestyle. Now it's up to you to choose whether you want to be part of this amazing lifestyle or not.

It's not a one-size-fits-all prescription, and it's crucial to work with a dietitian to ensure you're getting essential nutrients while maintaining ketosis. There's promising research on the benefits of the ketogenic diet for many conditions, but some people can't keep it up for the long haul, plus the long-term effects are poorly understood. If you decide to go keto, work with a dietitian to help you create a nutrition plan.
The real question is, do you want to feel great, be more energetic, and overall healthier? And guess what, after a bit of a transition you'll never have to give it much thought again. It'll be second nature and a true lifestyle - not a fad and not a diet.

ABOUT THE AUTHOR

My name is Glenis Graham and I have been striving to always do my best at almost everything I do. Taking care of myself and looking my best is no exception. As far back as I can remember as a child everyone encourages success.

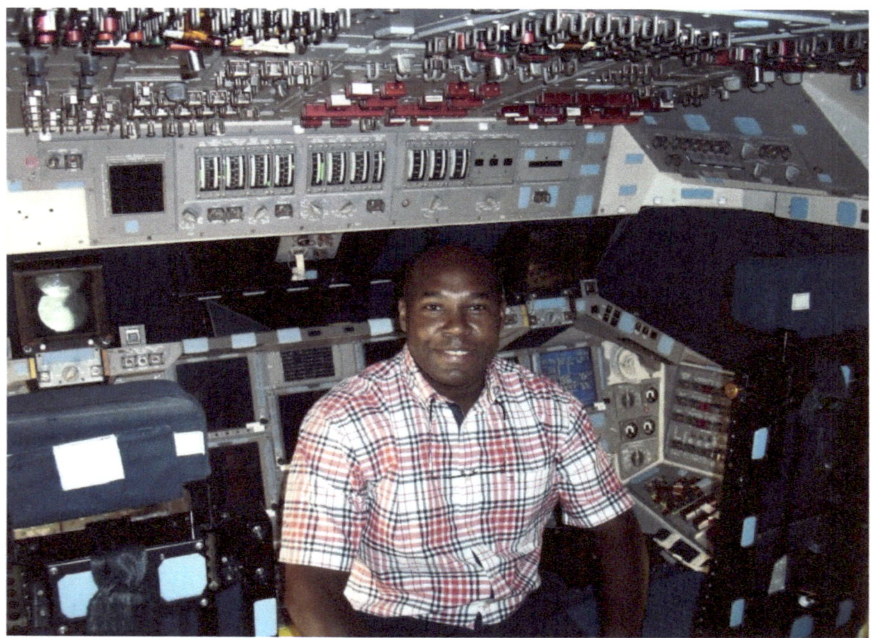

So, here is where I share with you why I wrote this Maxx Ketosis Guide. I tried the ketosis diet and found that it to be extremely helpful in more ways than just losing weight, however, once you get into ptosis it's very difficult to maintain and be consistent. I looked all over for a detailed and helpful guide to assist, but to my surprise, there was nothing that I found helpful. So wanted to write down some of the things that I found to be important in maximizing my ketosis experience.

9 798541 920758